IT'S

WELLNESS, NATURALLY

Dr. Finker Reveals the Healing Benefits of Naturopathic Medicine

Dr. Jillian Finker, N.D.

Disclaimer

The information contained in this book is not medical advice. Be sure to seek your doctor for any kind of treatment. Please note that the laws for naturopathic treatment vary from state to state.

No action should be taken based solely on the contents of this book. Readers should consult appropriate health professionals on any matter relating to their health and well-being.

The information and opinions provided here are believed to be accurate and sound, based on the best information available to the author at this time. Readers who fail to consult appropriate health authorities assume the risk of any injuries. This book is not responsible for errors or omissions.

By reading this book, you assume all risks associated with using the advice contained within, with a full understanding that you, solely, are responsible for anything that may occur as a result of putting this information into action in any way, regardless of your interpretation of the advice.

You further agree that the author cannot be held responsible in any way for the success or failure of your business as a result of the information presented below. It is your responsibility to conduct your own due diligence regarding the safe and successful operation of your business, if you intend to apply any of our information in any way to your business operations.

Table of Contents

Dedication

I would like to thank my parents, Paul and Mindy Finker, who introduced me to the powers of naturopathic medicine at the early age of eight. I am so grateful for their unconditional love and support.

Also, I am thankful for the rest of my wonderful family, my colleagues and friends who have constantly supported me in all of my endeavors throughout the years; you know who you are.

Acknowledgments

I would like to dedicate this book to all of the patients out there who continuously show me how simple changes can transform lives into amazing journeys... Thank you for reminding me over and over again how wonderful life is and how magnificent it can be. Thank you.

Introduction

How I Got Here from There

Congratulations! The fact that you are reading these words indicates that you care about your health and that you want to feel great! Or perhaps you have a loved one in need of hope. Either way, you have come to the right place.

In my practice, I see a wide variety of patients at my clinics. I also treat an even greater selection of patients around the world via phone, email and Skype. I encounter patients with many different ideas about naturopathic medicine. Some patients discovered me on their own after being disappointed by traditional medical approaches. Others have sought me out as the first step in improving their well being. Still others may have been dragged in by a spouse or loved one. Yet, they all leave with hope.

There have been exciting advances in recent years in both traditional medical practices and procedures, and naturopathic treatments. There are patients who have excellent results with a traditional approach, others who fare better with a naturopathic approach, and still others who find the combination of both traditional and naturopathic treatments to be the most effective.

My intention in writing this book is to dispel the many myths about naturopathic medicine and to answer any questions you may have so that you can make an informed decision about the best way to approach your own healthcare.

Whether you're interested in naturopathic medicine because you've been struggling with your health, seeking ways to maintain your current health as you mature, or you are in the position of advising a loved one, I welcome you to the wonderful world of naturopathic medicine.

Why did you choose to become a naturopathic physician?

I've been asked this question many times by relatives, colleagues in the medical profession and patients. The answer is simple—because it changed my life.

I was eight years old when I started suffering from asthma attacks. I often felt like I was trying to breathe through a straw, and it was petrifying. I was sure I was going to suffocate each time I had an attack.

My family physician had prescribed an inhaler, which helped at first, but only for a little while. Next was a medication often used for respiratory conditions, but the "cure" was almost as bad as the ailment. My asthma got better, but I felt terrible: I was so anxious, I felt as if I had been given high doses of sugary snacks. I couldn't sleep and I kept my parents up night after night. Perhaps that was the impetus for my parents to seek alternative care!

My mother found a chiropractor practicing natural medicine. He did testing for food allergies and placed me on a strict diet. It wasn't easy with my friends making fun of me at birthday parties: I was eating my tasteless natural carob bars while they had cake. But in a few months, my asthma disappeared and I was able to play the sports I loved with the neighborhood kids, and sleep peacefully at night—no medication necessary!

So that was the start of my interest in a natural approach to health. But it wasn't until my senior year of college that my future was formed.

I had been placed on birth control pills by a local gynecologist to control the hormonal imbalances that had caused incapacitating cramping every month. They worked to regulate my cycle and heal the cramping, but I started to experience frightening abdominal pains. My gynecologist disagreed with my suggestion that the pain was being caused by the birth control pills, and I received a battery of tests, including a CAT scan. Everything came back negative: no explanation, just continued pain.

This time, it was my father who suggested I seek out a chiropractor who was also a practitioner of natural medicine. After some tests, he concluded that I should stop the birth control pills, and sure enough, after I did, the pain went away. He was then able to correct my hormonal imbalances with diet and supplements, which caused me to become a renewed believer in natural medicine, forever changing my life.

Just before this event, I had been considering my career as a health care practitioner and was interested in becoming a D.O. or a chiropractor. But this man who had (in my eyes) just performed a miracle, said that what I really wanted was to be a naturopath. Then he proceeded to tell me that he was enrolled in a school to become a licensed naturopathic doctor.

My mother, a registered nurse, offered her advice as well: "You'll never be satisfied as a traditional medical doctor; you will want to be able to spend more time with your patients," she said.

I began extensive research into the field of naturopathic medicine and the curriculums available for licensing (this was before the days of "Google Search!"). Finally, I was clear on my life's mission and the program that would get me started on my path. I attended the Southwest College of Naturopathic Medicine in Tempe, Arizona, and obtained my license in 2003.

What kinds of patients do you see?

Naturopathic doctors are primary care doctors, so my main focus after passing the board exams was family medicine.

I've been able to help a wide range of patients in my practice who present with conditions ranging from infertility to migraines, to diabetes and cardiac disease. I've treated everything from chronic ear infections in pediatric patients, to severe anxiety in elderly patients. I've also treated both men and women with hormonal imbalances.

Do you specialize in any specific conditions?

I chose to take extra steps to specialize my practice, based mainly on my own experiences as a young woman. In addition to my required training, I took extra coursework in order to have a focus in women's health, hormonal imbalances and gastrointestinal problems. Consequently, I treat many women for fibroids, infertility, menopause and thyroid issues. I also treat patients with blood sugar issues, adrenal gland problems and other hormonal imbalances, including those that often result in anxiety and depression.

Can you really help me with my specific problem?

Many patients who come to one of my clinics have been seen previously by a variety of primary care doctors and/or specialists. It's not uncommon for them to be discouraged and doubtful of the possibility for improvement, as they may have been told that "there's just nothing that can be done" about their disease. Many think that they're always going to feel sick, so they often ask me, *"Have you handled this situation before? Can you really help me with my specific problem?"*

My response is that I have many years of experience treating a wide variety of disorders, and I can help just about any patient who walks into my office. If I assess that I am not the best practitioner to help a given patient, I will refer them to another doctor who specializes in the kind of treatment they need.

What do you do if you don't have experience treating my health problem?

There are rare occasions when a patient presents with a condition that I've never treated, or have treated infrequently. The beauty of naturopathic medicine is that it is based on sound principles including the interplay of diet, exercise and lifestyle. Therefore, they apply to almost any health problem I encounter.

In addition, there are many forums I use on a regular basis to communicate with different naturopaths across the United States. I am lucky enough to have wonderful connections with my colleagues, so I can find out what they use to treat their patients. I also have access to several databases filled with research studies to confirm the effectiveness of both traditional and naturopathic treatments that have worked for other patients.

What can I expect when I come to your office?

My goal with any new patient is to obtain as much information as I can about her current situation, including symptoms, medications, medical test results, diet and lifestyle. I also conduct a detailed assessment of previous treatments, obtain a comprehensive medical history, and perform a comprehensive naturopathic examination. I want to know everything that could be impacting a patient's current state of health in order to assess the potential to bring immediate relief, as well as produce sustainable long-term results.

You may be surprised at some of the questions I ask. Do you crave chocolate? If so, perhaps you need a magnesium supplement. Do you remember your dreams? If not, you may be deficient in B vitamins. Are you frustrated that you can't lose weight even though your thyroid has tested in the normal range? Perhaps it is working sub-clinically, or there are other contributing factors to weight gain, such as elevated estrogen levels.

Even more important for some patients is the assessment of how they're feeling emotionally. If you've never been to a naturopath, you might be skeptical. Or perhaps you're frightened because you've already tried many approaches unsuccessfully. Feeling depressed or anxious is also natural when your health has been compromised in some way. But you're not alone!

My initial appointment with patients lasts at least an hour so that I have a chance to get to know them and fully understand their concerns. Follow up appointments usually last 30–60 minutes and vary in frequency, depending on the severity of the patient's illness.

I prefer to space the scheduling of my patients so that there is minimal waiting time. I also ensure that the reception area is a peaceful environment for patients to relax before the visit. I also make myself available in between appointments to answer any questions that may surface. My goal is for my patients to be able to get in touch with me if necessary and to feel secure in the knowledge that I'm there for them.

A meticulous and thorough approach to each individual who comes through my door is the hallmark of my practice. Each patient is special to me and I experience great joy seeing what people are capable of when they feel their best!

How can I use this book?

I invite you to explore my world. I've provided a thorough overview of the naturopathic approach to health.

You'll find that many of the recommendations involve choices that are yours to make right now, tips that can help you feel and look younger.

In my experience, as long as the body is being cared for internally, it will automatically reflect in the outward appearance of any person. I've had patients telling me they feel 10–15 years younger after following my recommendations. Their freedom of movement increases as their pain decreases; they acquire a more active lifestyle, lose weight and feel happier overall.

This book is structured to answer your questions and help you make the best decision for obtaining and maintaining an optimum state of health and wellness so that you can experience all that life has to offer.

You can use this book in two ways:

1. Read the chapters in sequential order to obtain a full picture of naturopathic medicine: the training required for NDs, standard treatment approaches and patient testimonials.

2. Browse through the book and review the questions and answers integrated into each chapter. These are questions typically asked by patients considering a naturopathic medical approach to health. See what piques your interest.

There are also a number of articles and patient testimonials that may serve as the perfect answer to your questions and concerns.

I also invite you to visit my website: *www.drfinker.com* and to connect with me via *Facebook* and *LinkedIn*.

Here's to your health!
—*Dr. Jillian Finker*

Chapter 1

The Naturopathic Doctor

What is a naturopathic doctor?

A naturopathic doctor, also known as an ND, is a primary care physician who is also an expert in alternative medicine. Naturopathic doctors are considered to be general practitioners who are capable of treating many healthcare problems, including all aspects of family health from prenatal care to geriatric care.

Naturopathic doctors value the concept of "holism" (emphasizing the importance of the body as a whole) and they treat the body as an integrated, complex system. They go beyond the patient's superficial symptoms to discover their underlying cause. This complete and thorough approach affords them the opportunity to heal the underlying cause of the patient's symptoms, consequently bringing the whole body back to health.

How are they trained?

Contrary to some popular beliefs, naturopathic doctors receive extensive education and training in alignment with that received by traditional medical doctors. Not only do they have to complete a four-year undergraduate program

1

of pre-medical training, and comply with admission requirements comparable to (and sometimes greater than) those of regular medical schools, they are also trained in natural therapeutics. This allows them the opportunity to treat the body holistically.

Undergraduate training includes classes in botany, psychology, anatomy, physiology, organic chemistry and physics. Naturopathic medical college requires another four years of graduate-level medical classes, including anatomy, neurology, cardiology, biochemistry, microbiology, minor surgery, radiology, pathology and immunology. Diagnostic processes and clinical rotations are a standard part of naturopathic medical training, as they are with traditional medical school training. Naturopathic doctors receive 1,200 hours of clinical training along with 4,100 hours of didactic training.

In addition to standard medical school training, the curriculum for naturopathic doctors includes training in nutrition, botanical medicine, homeopathy, acupuncture, hydrotherapy and many other natural techniques not traditionally offered in regular medical schools. Naturopathic doctors are then required to pass board exams very similar to standard medical school board exams, resulting in a license as a naturopathic doctor. After achieving licensure, a doctor can then be referred to as a naturopathic doctor (ND), a naturopathic medical doctor (NMD) or a naturopathic physician. Both the Department of Education and the Carnegie Institute classify the ND degree as a first-professional degree under Doctorate-Professional (clinical), on par with MD and DO degrees.

Do they specialize?

After passing the board exams, naturopathic doctors are qualified as primary care physicians, so their main focus is often family medicine. Some naturopathic doctors choose to pursue additional specialized training in order to become board-certified in other fields, including cardiology, endocrinology, gynecology and pediatrics.

What kinds of conditions can they treat?

A naturopathic doctor can help a patient with any condition that would require the attention of a primary care doctor. They treat conditions ranging from migraines and the flu, to sore throats and ear infections, as well as many other acute problems. They can also treat chronic conditions such as diabetes and cardiac disease, and hormone-related problems such as infertility, menopause, osteoporosis, ovarian cysts, fibroids, hypo- and hyperthyroidism, and adrenal gland diseases. An ND can also treat a variety of gastrointestinal problems, ranging from simple gas-induced bloating to acid reflux and irritable bowel syndrome.

In addition to these physical conditions, naturopathic doctors can also help patients with emotional problems, such as anxiety, depression, fatigue and insomnia. The overall scope of an ND is quite extensive—they can address almost any health concern. When appropriate, they will also partner with traditional medical doctors— both primary care and specialists—to meet the needs of their patients.

Chapter 2

The Naturopathic Difference

What is the difference between a naturopathic doctor and a traditional medical doctor?

The difference between a naturopathic doctor and a traditional medical doctor can best be understood by examining the difference between a "symptomatic" versus a "holistic" approach to health.

The Symptomatic Approach to Health

When a traditional medical doctor is presented with a symptomatic patient, he prescribes the appropriate medications to alleviate the patient's symptoms and that may be where the consult ends. Some traditional medical practitioners do not look deeper into the actual cause of the symptoms, so their approach is considered only "symptomatic" in nature.

The Holistic Approach to Health

Naturopathic doctors are trained to treat the patient as a whole, integrated person. In other words, they take the entire body into consideration, with all of its organ systems. They view the body as an integrated, complex system, where a disease in one part automatically has an impact on all of the other parts.

Besides taking the time to carefully and fully assess the root cause of the patient's problem, NDs speak and understand the language of conventional medicine. Naturopathic doctors diagnose diseases, and they bring a whole new arsenal of treatments and insights to the patient.

This is considered a "holistic" approach versus simply a "symptomatic" approach. Naturopathic doctors routinely look beyond the patients' surface symptoms to find and treat the underlying cause of these symptoms. By identifying the root cause of the issue rather than simply solving the superficial problems presented by the patient, NDs are often able to provide sustainable, long-lasting solutions for the patient's overall health, resulting in a level of well-being previously unknown to the patient.

It should be noted that providing symptomatic relief is extremely important, and that some conditions can be eradicated with this approach. However, in general, naturopathic doctors prefer to take a proactive, strategic approach to wellness: instead of waiting for a disease to emerge, NDs work to prevent the cause of the disease before it happens.

Can you give me an example of the difference between the symptomatic and holistic approach?

Consider a patient who is suffering from acid reflux, a disorder that results in a burning pain in the upper stomach. A naturopathic doctor would use some of the same techniques and diagnostic criteria used by a traditional medical doctor: she would examine the abdomen, take stool and blood samples, and send the samples out to a laboratory to determine the underlying cause of the acid reflux. The ND might also recommend certain prescription medications, similar to those recommended by a traditional physician.

However, the real difference in the naturopathic approach is in its focus on taking the next step to discover the root cause of the disease. For example, if no pathology was found in this acid reflux patient, a typical medical doctor might end the consult with the prescription medication. Unfortunately, the medication often does nothing other than mask the pain.

Naturopathic doctors, on the other hand, look closely to determine what is actually *causing* the pain. Next steps might include additional testing, including a more expansive stool panel, comprehensive blood work, or other tests to determine if the patient has too much or too little acid in the digestive tract. They might also run tests to see if the patient has *dysbiosis* (an overgrowth of pathogenic bacteria in the gastrointestinal tract and an undergrowth of healthy bacteria like acidophilus), as well as decreased enzyme production, or inflammation. When they finally discover the pathology underlying the symptoms, naturopathic physicians will treat it accordingly, in order to heal the disease itself and bring the patient lasting relief.

In the example of our acid reflux patient, the underlying cause of the patient's stomach pain could be food allergies. When a patient consumes a food she is allergic to, the stomach lining can become irritated, resulting in a burning sensation. So whenever a patient with a food allergy or intolerance consumes an allergenic food, she will experience a burning pain in her stomach.

In this example, instead of merely administering an antacid or a medication that decreases the amount of acid production, the naturopathic doctor would address the root cause of the problem. An ND would recommend that the patient should simply abstain from eating the offending foods. She would provide a protocol that would heal the gut lining with herbs and other nutrients. Also, she would normalize the immune system so the patients may be able to eventually tolerate the offending foods. Thus, a naturopathic approach would result in a *solution* to the medical condition itself, rather than providing a mere "Band-Aid" to the original symptoms.

Chapter 3

The Naturopathic Examination

What can I expect in terms of a physical examination and laboratory testing?

As discussed in the first chapter, naturopathic doctors are trained in the same manner as medical doctors, especially in the basic medical sciences. They are also highly trained in performing comprehensive physical examinations. They examine the different parts of the body, looking for signs that may point to an underlying pathology. There are many subtle signs in the body that point to pathology, and naturopathic doctors are specifically trained to identify and treat them accordingly.

In addition to conducting thorough physical examinations, NDs use laboratory tests as an aid to the diagnosis and treatment of patients. They are trained to use imaging modalities such as CAT scans, X-rays and MRIs in the same way as standard M.D.'s. However, they may view the results from these diagnostic tools in a different way than is typical of a traditional medical approach.

Can you give me an example?

Let us follow the process that a naturopathic doctor would take for a patient with a thyroid imbalance who is suffering from fatigue, weight gain and depression.

It is common practice for both a naturopathic doctor and a traditional medical doctor to order a blood test when presented with a patient who may have a thyroid imbalance. However, these two doctors will often view the results of this same blood test in a very different manner. In fact, blood test levels that show up as "normal" on traditional lab work may actually be on the lower range of normal, and the patient may still have symptoms. For example, if someone has a thyroid stimulating hormone (TSH) level of 3.0 and they have symptoms, a naturopathic doctor will support the thyroid even though it is within "normal" limits. This can then cause the patient's problematic thyroid symptoms to disappear.

A traditional medical doctor may check just one parameter related to these test results, like the thyroid stimulating hormone (TSH) levels. They often look at this parameter to see if their patient needs to be prescribed a pharmaceutical like *Synthroid* to normalize thyroid function.

A naturopathic doctor, on the other hand, will usually run a comprehensive thyroid panel, which includes many different markers. They want to see the complete picture of the patient's thyroid function to determine if their thyroid problem is due to nutritional deficiencies that require supplementation.

Many patients who take *Synthroid* are still overweight, and some may be suffering from other problems associated with a poorly functioning thyroid. Thus, looking only at the TSH level may not be as helpful as it could be: Patients can have a normal TSH level and yet still have thyroid problems. That is why a naturopathic doctor will usually run several other tests to determine whether the *Synthroid* is working optimally or whether other modalities are needed to normalize the thyroid and relieve the symptoms.

What are some other tests used by naturopathic doctors?

Aside from blood work, naturopathic doctors often use other diagnostic tools, such as saliva and urine tests. These tests often identify subtle problems in the body that are missed by blood work alone. As shown in the previous example, a patient may have "normal" blood test results, and yet still have hormonal imbalances. Even when the results are examined carefully with different parameters that include the low or high end of normal, blood work can only show a momentary "snapshot" of what is actually going on inside the body.

For example, blood work that measures a patient's progesterone levels would only reflect physiologic function in the body for that particular day. Salivary and urinary tests, on the other hand, provide a picture of how the levels may be changing over time. These tests can be done at home at the patient's convenience, and then progesterone levels can be measured over the course of an entire month. In this way, a naturopathic doctor can get a clear picture of the patient's hormone levels for that entire monthly cycle.

Naturopathic physicians also request tests to back up, support or augment other tests. For example, thermography is an excellent diagnostic tool for breast cancer or a person's predisposition to develop breast cancer. When these thermographic findings are coupled with other tests, such as mammography and breast ultrasound, their diagnostic value increases. Thus, thermography can be a good adjunct to the diagnosis and early detection of breast cancer.

In summary, naturopathic doctors combine the wisdom of nature with the rigors of modern science. Steeped in traditional healing methods, principles and practices, naturopathic medicine focuses on holistic, proactive prevention and comprehensive diagnosis and treatment. By using protocols that minimize the risk of harm, naturopathic doctors help facilitate the body's inherent ability to restore and maintain optimal health. It is the naturopathic doctor's role to identify and remove barriers to good health by helping to create a healing internal and external environment.

Chapter 4

Nutrition, Herbs and Homeopathy

How will my naturopathic doctor help me to heal?

Naturopathic doctors use many different modalities to bring the body back to health, including nutrition, homeopathy, botanicals or herbs, supplements, and even lifestyle changes.

Eating Your Way to Good Health

NDs consider clinical nutrition to be one of the most important healing modalities. In fact, the use of food to maintain health and treat illnesses is often considered to be the foundation of naturopathic medicine.

Food and nutrition are fundamental to the human body's ability to heal itself. Thus, eating the right type and the right amount of food can have a dramatic impact upon your health. There are many scientific studies supporting this premise, which show that many medical problems can be effectively treated with food and nutritional supplements, bypassing many of the side effects encountered with prescription medications.

Can you give me an example of how food can heal or hurt me?

Patients with significant hormonal imbalances, weight gain, abdominal bloating and other health problems suddenly felt better simply after removing processed soy from their diet. How is this possible? Soy can be very irritating to the gastrointestinal tract, and it can also cause thyroid and female hormonal imbalances. As a result, when soy was removed from their diets, these patients often experienced sudden and dramatic improvements in their health. That is exactly how a small change in diet can bring about big changes in the overall health of a patient.

Herbs/Botanicals

Herbal or botanical treatments are another modality frequently used by naturopathic doctors. Herbs are used to bring the body back to balance. They are powerful medicines, and when used correctly, are proven to be nontoxic and can be as or more effective than pharmaceuticals.

Herbs are administered in many different forms, such as teas, powders and extracts. Naturopathic doctors are trained to determine which method of intake is best suited for a particular patient.

Does homeopathy really work?

Naturopathic doctors also use homeopathy to help heal the body. Homeopathy entails using diluted substances to cure illnesses. It is a system of medicine that has been around for over two hundred years, and is considered one of the safest ways to treat a wide array of illnesses.

The main principle of homeopathy is based on the idea of the dilution of different substances, which greatly reduces the chances of unpleasant side effects. However, because these medications are so highly diluted, people often suspect that the healing power of homeopathy is just based on a "placebo effect"—a phenomenon in which a patient's symptoms are relieved simply because she believes in the treatment (the treatment actually contains an inactive substance).

While many consider this viewpoint to be true, homeopathic remedies have been shown to work countless times on infants and animals. These populations have no concept of "medicine," thus casting doubt on the placebo effect, and reinforcing the importance of homeopathy as a viable and effective treatment modality.

What is the difference between nutritionists, herbalists and homeopaths?

People often wonder if a naturopathic doctor is the same as a homeopathic doctor or a nutritionist. In fact, an ND could be considered both, because a naturopathic doctor is trained both in nutrition and homeopathy.

NDs are experts in utilizing nutrition, herbs and homeopathy to bring the body back to health, though their training is still firmly rooted in traditional medicine. Naturopathic doctors are trained to be physicians first, and they use their medical training to discern when and how to employ different modalities, such as homeopathy and nutrition.

For example, through symptom identification and blood tests, a naturopathic doctor can determine if a patient has an iron deficiency. After being diagnosed, the patient may be treated successfully with iron supplements, or may undergo further testing with a specific, very sensitive stool panel to determine whether the cause of the iron deficiency is an underlying parasitic infection. If a parasitic infection is found, it can then be treated with herbs, vitamins or even pharmaceuticals, if necessary. Therefore, a naturopathic doctor can be considered a nutritionist, herbalist *and* homeopath... in addition to being a highly trained medical doctor.

Chapter 5

Lifestyle Modification

What is meant by "lifestyle modification?"

One of the greatest benefits that patients enjoy from working with a naturopathic physician is the development of a close patient-doctor relationship through effective communication. Naturopathic doctors are trained to actively listen and counsel patients, which is critical to the healing process. Through active dialogue with their patients, naturopathic doctors can recognize mental attitudes or emotional stressors that are contributing to their patient's illness. They can also discover what aspect of a patient's lifestyle may be affecting his health, and subsequently give the patient advice to help him modify certain habits and activities. The result? Happier, healthier patients.

Lifestyle Modification as Part of Preventive Medicine

Most diseases of the human body have a contributing lifestyle component—an underlying cause connected to the way we live. Heart disease, diabetes and even

17

cancer can often be prevented by simply living a healthier lifestyle.

For instance, stress has been implicated as a contributing factor to the development of heart disease. In fact, studies have shown that most people have heart attacks on Mondays—the most stressful day of the work week.

Other studies have shown that the longer someone drives in traffic during their daily commute, the more likely they are to have a heart attack, which is probably due to both stress and pollution.

Also, if someone lives on a busy street, they are more likely to develop rheumatoid arthritis—a disease of the joints that can be very debilitating for patients. This is probably due to the pollution that these people are exposed to.

On the flip side, it has been shown that exercise (a positive lifestyle habit) is actually more effective than taking antidepressants to treat depression. And the list goes on and on…

The bottom line is that diseases are all linked to our lifestyle and daily living habits. So if you want to prevent certain diseases, your first steps should focus on lifestyle modification.

How do I go about making the right lifestyle modifications?

Lifestyle modification simply involves two factors: (1) making the right decision and (2) sticking with that decision. Everyone has the ability to make choices; and the choices that we make can lead up to the path of good health or down to the path of disease. In order to make the best decision for one's health, it is important to be well-informed about the various choices and the consequences of those choices.

This is where naturopathic doctors can play an important role. They can help patients fine-tune their dietary and lifestyle choices. Educated patients are empowered patients, and they can make the choices that are beneficial to their health.

Can I prevent a hereditary disease?

Many patients with relatives who have certain hereditary or familial diseases, including cancer, diabetes, thyroid issues and other diseases that "run in the family," believe that they are genetically predisposed to an illness and there is nothing they can do to avoid contracting a certain condition.

The good news is that if a patient has a relative with a particular disease or health condition, it does not *guarantee* that he is going to develop the same problem. In fact, even though these diseases may have strong genetic components, there are <u>many</u> causes that lead to the development of a particular disease—genetics are only one of those factors, and should never be thought of as the ultimate determinant in these situations.

For example, there are many case studies of identical twins wherein one manifests a given disease while the other does not. This indicates the importance that both our internal and external environments play in disease development. So, even if someone is at risk for certain hereditary diseases, he still has control over many contributing factors (such as diet, environment, and physical activity), and he may not necessarily develop the disease.

What can I do to prevent the onset of a hereditary disease?

If patients have a strong family history of a disease such as diabetes, they can prevent its development by making specific healthy changes. In fact, studies have shown that the development of diabetes can be triggered by chromium deficiency. Therefore, certain patients can help to prevent the onset of diabetes by taking chromium supplements. Patients can also maintain a healthy blood sugar level by frequently eating small meals that include protein. Minor changes such as these can have a major impact on diabetes prevention.

What about preventing heart disease?

Even if someone has a strong family history of heart disease, she can take steps to prevent it by maintaining a healthy diet. This includes avoiding foods rich in trans-fats, and eating foods which are high in "good cholesterol." Exercising regularly and reducing stress levels are also proven ways to maintain a healthy heart.

What can I do to prevent cancer?

There are some preventive measures shown to reduce the risk of cancer that can be easily implemented. For instance, some studies have shown that artificial light at night (such as a night-light or a street lamp projecting light into a bedroom) can increase a patient's risk of developing cancer. If there are small, preventive measures that can be made today to reduce the risk of a disease like cancer for the long-term, why not give them a try?

In summary, even if a patient is genetically predisposed to develop a given disease or condition, it is never a guarantee that she will clinically manifest the disease. The good news is that people can make various small changes to their lifestyle to protect themselves from developing these hereditary diseases.

Chapter 6

Mind and Body Techniques

What is meant by the mind-body connection?

Naturopathic doctors use different mind-body techniques to bring the body back to health, because thoughts and emotions can have a dramatic physical effect on the body.

Can you give me an example of how my thoughts affect my body?

One of the best examples of how your thoughts can impact your body in a positive or negative way is the "chocolate cake study." In this study, it was found that if a person has strong negative thoughts when she is eating a piece of chocolate cake, it can actually lower the effectiveness of her body's immune system. Yet, if she thinks positively while eating this cake, her immunity remains unchanged. This is a good indication that what we feed our minds is just as important as what we feed our body.

How is the mind-body connection related to feelings, such as anxiety and depression?

Naturopathic physicians see many people on a daily basis who are experiencing some level of anxiety and/or depression even though they do not indicate it as their chief complaint. There is almost always a direct physical component that is contributing to these feelings.

Many physical conditions can bring on feelings of anxiety. For instance, if a patient has a blood sugar issue (especially low blood sugar), it can mimic the feeling of panic or anxiety. When blood sugar levels drop, the body releases cortisol to restore sugar levels to a normal level. Perhaps not coincidentally, cortisol is the same hormone that the body releases under stress. Consequently, patients with low blood sugar are often diagnosed with anxiety.

Naturopathic doctors seek to heal the underlying physical component related to blood sugar levels, and once the patient's levels are stabilized, the anxiety the patient was originally experiencing sometimes disappears completely. It is as if the mind is being healed through the healing of the body.

Patients who originally experienced such debilitating anxiety that they were not able to leave their homes are often able to lead very normal lives after treatment. For example, new mothers with postpartum depression, who previously experienced crying every day, are now able to experience happiness and emotional stability in their lives once they are diagnosed and treated properly.

Why didn't anyone else treat me appropriately for anxiety and depression?

Though this is not always the case, some traditional medical doctors may focus primarily on the symptoms presented by the patient rather than the subtle, underlying cause. They might prescribe anti-depressants and encourage their patients to see a therapist without addressing the true cause. Thus, some patients might walk away feeling as if the anxiety and depression are just in their head. They may not realize there is a physical connection.

Prescription treatment modalities can be very effective, particularly with patients who have debilitating anxiety or depression and need immediate relief of their symptoms. However, these treatments only address the symptoms of the patient's problem, and do not target the underlying cause.

The goal of the naturopathic doctor is to bring their patients back to a state of optimal health, by supporting both the body and the mind, and by addressing any contributing physical components of their illnesses.

Chapter 7

Nutraceuticals and Food Supplements

What are "nutraceuticals?"

Nutraceuticals, a term derived from the words "nutrition" and "pharmaceuticals," pertains to a group of products that are isolated or purified from food. These products include vitamins and minerals like iron, magnesium and zinc, which are commonly used as food supplements. These products are often used by naturopathic doctors to correct nutritional imbalances or deficiencies in the body.

Why can't I get what I need from my food?

NDs are often asked why nutraceuticals are needed if they are just derived from food in the first place. Understandably, patients question why they may need food supplements in addition to a healthy diet. The answer can be found in the amount of vitamins and minerals that our bodies are able to derive from our daily diet. It is very difficult to get all of the nutrients that are needed from food alone. For example, you would need to eat almost eight cups of kale a day to get the amount of magnesium necessary for optimal health. Obviously, most patients are not willing or able to consume such high quantities of vegetables. Even if a patient was willing to take on such a strict eating regimen, it would still take the body quite a while to build up various nutrients. So it would take longer for the body to heal solely through dietary changes. Consequently, most naturopathic doctors recommend various food supplements to their patients.

How do I know what supplements I need?

Naturopathic physicians are highly trained to assess which nutrients are lacking in a patient's diet, and they only recommend supplements after assessing if there is truly a nutrient deficiency.

As an example, there are a number of scientific studies indicating that zinc supplements can decrease the severity and duration of colds. Yet there are also contradictory articles that say zinc supplements have no beneficial effects for the common cold.

Now which is true? Well, zinc happens to be effective only if the patient has low levels of zinc. For those patients with adequate zinc levels, taking zinc supplements will not provide additional relief.

The zinc example proves how important it is for doctors to assess patients prior to prescribing supplements. Naturopathic doctors excel at assessing and treating patients with nutritional deficiencies, and they ensure that patients do not waste their money on supplements they do not need.

How does my naturopathic doctor determine the dosage of my supplements?

Naturopathic doctors use a myriad of techniques to determine the correct dosage of supplements. For example, they look at the severity of the illness, the weight of the patient, markers in blood work, etc. They also look at scientific studies that offer dosage recommendations for various supplements.

However, a unique aspect of nutritional supplements is that they are "modulating" in nature. In other words, regardless of the dosage prescribed, they can help regulate various hormone and fat levels in the body. This capacity makes them very different from pharmaceuticals. For example, if a patient is taking fish oil, it normalizes the body's cholesterol level regardless of whether the initial level of cholesterol was high or low. So the end result is the same: normal cholesterol levels. In fact, prescribing the correct dosage with nutraceuticals is so much easier than prescribing pharmaceuticals. Nutraceuticals are so effective in modulating the human body that dosage and administration are much easier to determine.

Can supplements heal my condition?

To better illustrate the healing effects of supplements, consider the following example:

Several patients present with debilitating migraines — they are in horrible pain and they have not been able to do anything about it.

For these patients, the solution can be as simple as treating a magnesium deficiency. An adequate dose of magnesium can bring almost immediate pain relief. Patients are relieved and amazed that their terrible headaches have been eradicated by a simple supplement such as magnesium.

The amazing thing about the human body is that it can become quite ill simply from the lack of certain nutrients. Adding a certain food supplement to the diet can dramatically improve a patient's overall health. After a few days or weeks of simple supplementation, patients are sometimes relieved of their pain, healed of their disease, and feeling great about their bodies. It is extremely rewarding for patients—and their doctors—to see that they are able to create results like this simply by making a small nutritional adjustment.

I take a multivitamin every day—isn't that enough?

Many patients take multivitamins as part of a daily routine. However, while multivitamins are a good source of nutrition, their nutrient levels are often insufficient to bring the body back to optimal health or to cure diseases. They have beneficial effects, but they are not "silver bullets."

How do I know if the supplements I am taking are of good quality and are supporting my body?

Properly caring for your body is analogous to caring for your car. Cars filled with high-quality fuel run very smoothly. Cars filled with low-grade fuel run poorly. If you are taking poor-quality supplements, it is like trying to drive a car filled with low-grade fuel. On the other hand, if you are taking high-quality supplements, it is like driving a luxury vehicle powered by premium fuel. Your body is your own personal luxury vehicle and you want to keep it running at a high level of performance throughout your life. Thus, it makes sense to invest in high-quality vitamin supplements.

While it is certainly possible to find quality supplements in many health food stores, it is often difficult for the average consumer to assess the quality of supplements being sold in retail outlets. A naturopathic doctor has expertise in this area, and can easily assess the quality of any vitamins and/or supplements to determine if they are of value and if they are necessary to take on a daily basis.

Too often, patients unknowingly choose low-quality supplements that contain fillers and/or artificial colors and flavors. Also, cheap fish oils can be full of heavy metals, and they can even be rancid. It is hard for the untrained patient to discern the quality of the plethora of choices in many "health food" stores.

As a result, a Naturopathic Physician may recommend certain brands of supplements that they have evaluated as safe and effective, products that will help their patients achieve optimal results. They often make recommendations based on their own experience and research. They also suggest the brands they have seen work clinically, or possibly brands they have used themselves. They prescribe these supplements because they know that they have healed patients many times in their practice.

How does my naturopathic doctor know which supplements are best for me?

Naturopathic doctors use a set of criteria to ensure that the supplements they recommend are logical, effective, and safe for use. For instance:

1. Before prescribing a supplement, your physician will understand the various studies that support the use of that specific supplement. It is important to know whether the supplement will be well-absorbed within the body, and will actually be helpful for the various health conditions for which it is being recommended in the first place. It is also critical to make sure that the supplement does not contain any heavy metals or additives.

2. Many NDs will recommend supplements that they have personally taken themselves, because it helps to experience first-hand the results they are able to create in their body before they recommend them to their patients. Obviously, they cannot do this for all of the supplements they prescribe to their patients, but they will at the very least be familiar with the supplement manufacturer.

3. NDs only recommend supplements which have been proven to create positive results for their patients. They want to personally observe an improvement in their patients' symptoms, blood tests or other therapeutic markers. If they are going to use a relatively new supplement, they will often confer with their colleagues to make sure that other practitioners have used it and have seen consistent results in their own patient population.

In addition to these three important standards, your naturopathic doctor may also apply other precautionary measures when selecting supplements. For example, she will make sure that the supplements do not include any genetically modified ingredients, and that the supplements contain exactly what is stated on the bottle's label. Doctors also ensure the supplements are kept at room temperature or in the refrigerator when appropriate, and are safe and effective for patient use.

Most naturopathic doctors also have a strict policy about returned supplements. They do not put them "back on the shelf" because they cannot determine that those returned supplements were kept in a proper environment after they were purchased. In addition, they may recommend to their patients who buy supplements online that they get their supplements directly from the manufacturing company. This is the safest policy for many reasons, one of which is to avoid legal issues arising from online retailers selling supplements illegally. For instance, there have been cases where retailers put labels on containers that were different from the actual product. However, these issues can be avoided if you buy directly from the manufacturer.

Take advantage of the wealth of knowledge and expertise your ND can offer you in terms of choosing the right supplements and the right brands to maintain optimal health as well as to get the most value for your money.

Chapter 8

Pharmaceuticals and Prescription Medications

Do naturopathic doctors prescribe pharmaceuticals to treat their patients?

Pharmaceuticals are chemical substances prescribed by physicians to treat medical conditions and diseases. They may be obtained as OTC (over-the-counter) medications or prescription medications: licensed medicines that are regulated by legislation to require a medical prescription before they can be obtained. The primary difference between pharmaceuticals and natural products like herbs and supplements lies in the nature of the body's response.

In most cases, the human body does not recognize pharmaceuticals as anything but foreign chemicals. This is because they are synthetically made in a lab and the molecular structure is different from anything the human body has experienced before. This explains why naturopathic doctors rarely use pharmaceuticals or prescription medications as first-line therapy. NDs will usually try natural products like supplementation and homeopathic remedies first when appropriate before they consider recommending pharmaceuticals.

Are naturopathic doctors allowed to prescribe pharmaceuticals?

In cases where pharmaceuticals are necessary to treat the patient, naturopathic doctors are likely to be able to prescribe them based upon the policies of the state in which they practice. The ability of NDs to prescribe pharmaceuticals can vary from state to state. This is because "prescription rights," the right to administer pharmaceuticals to patients, is not granted to naturopathic doctors in every state in the U.S. (due to the misconceptions previously described about the training required for NDs). However, policies are changing in states on a regular basis, and more and more states are granting naturopathic doctors full prescription rights since all NDs are required to be fully trained on how to utilize pharmaceuticals.

All naturopathic physicians have the ability to recommend the right medications based upon their diagnosis even if they are not always allowed to prescribe them. However, in these cases, naturopathic doctors often work with traditional medical doctors in order to administer pharmaceuticals to their patients. For more information about licensing and prescription rights, please visit Dr. Finker's website: *www.drfinker.com*

Why don't naturopathic doctors usually use pharmaceuticals as a first choice when treating patients?

Pharmaceuticals can be extremely effective under the right circumstances. They have the ability to save lives. However, many naturopathic doctors use them with discretion when appropriate because of their side effects. Also, as previously explained, NDs are committed to identifying the source of the disease or medical condition presented by the patient, and are careful not to use

34

pharmaceuticals for the sole purpose of symptomatic treatment.

Symptoms are important signals from the body that may herald a possible worsening of a patient's condition. They indicate that something is wrong with the body and are a message that the body is trying to heal itself. If prescription medications were used to address every patient's symptomatic complaints, the underlying cause of the disease may never be diagnosed or addressed.

Consider the analogy of a car "warning" light. When you see the "check engine light" in your car come on, it should raise a red flag that there could be something wrong with your engine. However, it would not help the situation to try to turn off that warning light by cutting the wires to the light on your dashboard. Instead, you should try to fix the engine itself, because that is why the light is coming on in the first place. If you fail to repair the underlying problem, you could very well find yourself stranded on the side of the road.

Similarly, if a patient has high cholesterol levels, it could be a signal from the body that there is a more complex medical issue involved. Thus, the patient could have subclinical hypothyroidism or chronic stress, which is causing his cholesterol levels to rise. To heal this patient completely, the underlying cause of the problem has to be diagnosed and treated accordingly rather than just removing the "warning signal" indicated by his symptoms.

For example, a patient's cholesterol levels can be effectively lowered in many cases through the use of a "cholesterol-lowering" pharmaceutical agent such as Lipitor. However, that would effectively remove the "warning light" that the body is flashing: namely, high cholesterol levels. By only addressing the cholesterol levels, it might appear that the situation is improving, but in fact the patient's condition may be progressing due to an underlying disease such as hypothyroidism, insulin resistance, high cortisol levels, and other various ailments.

Are you saying that I have to continue to suffer from my symptoms?

It should be reinforced that symptomatic relief is an important part of a patient's overall treatment plan and should not be postponed.

If a patient has severe back pain, it is important to relieve the pain as quickly as possible. Analgesics or painkillers are often necessary. Naturopathic doctors feel it is their duty to also discover the source of the pain, because the patient's "check-engine" light is flashing.

This principle can also be illustrated in the case of a patient with heartburn. When a patient experiences heartburn, his usual response is to take antacids to relieve the discomfort. However, it is very possible that the patient may have an *H. pylori* infection, which can be easily treated with antibiotics or various herbs. Instead of taking antacids for every episode of heartburn, patients can simply take antibiotics or herbs for a few weeks and the heartburn may go away forever.

It should now be apparent that it is very important to pay attention to the signals that our bodies provide. The symptoms that our bodies signal to us can provide us with clues to an underlying disease. Merely masking these clues with prescription drugs can be very dangerous, because our bodies can no longer tell us that the underlying cause of a condition is actually worsening.

Chapter 9

Supplement and Pharmaceutical Interactions

Could I have an adverse reaction by taking several supplements together?

With the increasing reports about adverse effects and drug interactions, many people are worried about taking different prescription drugs together. The idea of taking several pills simultaneously scares many patients, and they are right to express caution. Always check with your doctor or pharmacist before taking several pharmaceuticals together.

Supplement-Supplement Interactions

The good news is that supplements do *not* exhibit the negative interactions that are sometimes observed with the intake of multiple pharmaceuticals. This is because most supplements are food-based, so instead of interacting negatively, more often than not they complement one another.

For instance, it is not uncommon for naturopathic doctors to prescribe several supplements at once. They might recommend fish oil, multivitamins and Vitamin D for a given condition. Unlike pharmaceuticals, these supplements are all food-based, so when you take them together, it is similar to eating a meal. A typical meal contains multiple vitamins that you ingest simultaneously without experiencing any adverse effects, and the same is often true when patients take many supplements appropriately prescribed at the same time.

In addition to the inherent safety of supplements, the guidance of a naturopathic doctor ensures that any possible supplement interactions are avoided. In fact, NDs have the most extensive training in the medical field when it comes to assessing the proper dose and combination of given supplements to ensure there are no side effects.

Do supplements interact with medications?

Since many patients consult medical doctors before visiting a naturopathic doctor, it is very common for NDs to receive patients who are already taking prescription medications. The probability that these patients will be taking medications and supplements simultaneously is quite high. Because of that, naturopathic physicians have comprehensive training on potential interactions between supplements and pharmaceuticals. Thus, NDs are almost always more knowledgeable than any other practitioner about the adverse effects of combining pharmaceuticals and supplements.

The good news is that the interaction between medications and supplements can be very advantageous. For example, there can be synergistic effects between supplements and medications, whereby the supplements enhance the effects of the pharmaceutical in the body. As a result of this synergistic interaction, a patient is often able to decrease the dosage of their prescription drugs.

In addition, supplements can diminish the side effects of many pharmaceuticals.

Let's look again at the example of the cholesterol-lowering agent Lipitor. It can cause painful muscle aches in some patients because it depletes the bodys' store of CoQ10 (Coenzyme Q10), a naturally occurring antioxidant that helps to maintain proper cellular function. Knowing this, naturopathic doctors usually prescribe CoQ10 supplements to patients who are taking Lipitor in order to alleviate their muscle pain. However, NDs don't just stop there. Many naturopathic doctors will also advise their patients to make some dietary and lifestyle modifications, so that their cholesterol levels can be stabilized naturally. Most patients with high cholesterol levels can be treated effectively with supplementation, nutrition and lifestyle changes, and then they can eventually stop taking Lipitor altogether when appropriate.

Chapter 10

Side Effects

What kind of side effects can I expect with herbs and supplements?

When patients are presented with alternative treatment modalities such as herbs and supplements, it is understandable that they might be concerned about the possibility of side effects. However, almost all of the herbs and supplements used by naturopathic doctors have modulating effects, which means that they work by bringing your body back to balance. For example, when a diabetic patient with high blood sugar levels is prescribed herbs and supplements, her sugar level will decrease, but never beyond the normal levels. In contrast, prescription medications for diabetes, like insulin, can cause hypoglycemia or very low blood sugar, which can be very harmful for the patient.

Another positive aspect of supplements is that there is typically no danger of an overdose. For example, the worst thing that will probably happen if a patient takes too much of an appropriately prescribed supplement is an upset stomach. The body usually will simply pass the excess supplements naturally via bowel movements and urine.

In 2008, the Poison Control Center did a series of studies looking at the side effects of supplements. In that

41

study, they found no report of anyone dying from taking a dietary supplement—even without expert supervision. So supplements are quite safe, especially if you are in the care of an ND with many years of training in prescribing them to their patients.

Nevertheless, we should not consider herbs and supplements to be completely harmless in all cases. There are some patients who have allergic reactions to certain supplements because they may be allergic to the food that the supplement is comprised of. Fortunately, this kind of adverse reaction is rare, especially when an ND carefully screens her patients to gain a clear picture of which supplements will be beneficial and which should be avoided.

Keep in mind that supplements can also irritate the gastrointestinal tract of some patients who have sensitive stomachs. To prevent this from happening, a naturopathic physician will first heal the patient's pre-existing GI (gastrointestinal) conditions before she recommends certain supplements. So in essence, even if the alternative modalities have minor side effects, these effects can easily be prevented if you are in the care of a trained ND.

Chapter 11

Evidence-Based Therapeutics

Is there scientific evidence that naturopathic medicine is effective?

Naturopathic medicine is "evidence-based," meaning that almost every treatment is supported by a scientific foundation. There are many studies available that demonstrate this, including extensive research showing that alternative modalities cause little to no harm, and are effective in healing diseases.

Where can I find this scientific evidence?

PubMed is a free database available to the public; it serves as the medical doctor study search engine. Patients can access links to medical articles and journals, medical libraries and medical databases to learn about the safety and efficacy of almost every procedure and treatment included in a naturopathic doctor's practice.

Despite some misinformation about naturopathic medicine conveyed by the media, the totality of scientific evidence available on naturopathic medicine is overwhelmingly positive.

Naturopathic treatments are based on sound medical practices and researched scientific evidence. The results are all-inclusive, as patients are supported in creating positive changes in their health via nutrition, supplementation and healthy lifestyle choices. Symptoms can diminish and disappear as blood results and other test markers improve on a daily basis. Patients can be assured that the effectiveness of the naturopathic approach has been confirmed by studies that adhere to standard medical parameters.

Chapter 12

When to Visit a Naturopathic Doctor

When should I visit a naturopathic doctor?

Although a standard medical doctor is typically the first choice for a patient who is sick, he should also consider the benefits of seeing a naturopathic doctor as his "first stop" instead of as a last resort.

Naturopathic doctors are used to seeing at least one new patient daily who has been suffering from health problems for a long time. These patients have often incurred lots of time and spent lots of money on medications and treatments that were ineffective. Unfortunately, it is not uncommon to hear these patients tell their ND, "If this doesn't work, I don't know what I'm going to do."

The positive outcomes that come from healing very sick patients make them the most rewarding types of patients to treat. These patients often make drastic positive health changes in their lives, and their newfound health can seem almost miraculous in nature.

What kinds of patients have found relief?

Patients with chronic pain due to underlying conditions such as endometriosis, rheumatoid arthritis or osteoarthritis and fibromyalgia often seek help from a naturopathic doctor. These patients usually take pain relief medications (like aspirin or ibuprofen) every day, and yet they still experience severe chronic pain. However, as they are introduced to healthier habits such as regular exercise and diet supplementation, they almost always see dramatic healing changes. Many of them go on to live their daily lives pain free nearly forgetting about their previous chronic pain.

What about diseases that are hard to treat, such as chronic fatigue syndrome or severe infections?

Patients with chronic fatigue syndrome, who previously could not even get out of bed, may find themselves able to run around and play with their children after being treated by a naturopathic doctor. Children with chronic ear infections have been able to avoid surgery because their condition improved with natural therapeutics. Both the patient and the naturopathic doctor experience great satisfaction with the results that are possible with simple and natural treatments. Anyone who wants to experience an increase in well-being—a healthier body, optimal weight, longevity—can benefit from seeing a naturopathic doctor.

Chapter 13

Consulting with a Naturopathic Doctor

How much time will my naturopathic doctor spend with me?

Patients with a health problem who visit any kind of doctor usually experience a measure of anxiety, fear and concern over their illness. Naturally, they want a physician who is able to spend enough time with them to address all these issues. Consequently, patients are often frustrated with the increased brevity of medical consultations common in today's world. A ten-minute consultation is rarely enough to address all their concerns.

NDs are trained to understand that patients need quality time. Their patients may arrive feeling scared and confused. Many of them do not even understand the nature of their illnesses and are usually quite frustrated with the whole process. Many have been to different doctors before seeking the care of a naturopathic doctor, and some may have been told that their disease has no cure.

Naturopathic doctors receive training in counseling and therapy, and they make sure to spend enough time with each patient to ensure they have a comprehensive understanding of the patient's symptoms and circumstances. They are often able to reassure the patient that there are things they can do immediately to improve their health and heal their bodies.

In addition, many naturopathic doctors make it a personal practice to avoid overbooking their patients, as they do not want to rush their appointments or keep other patients waiting for too long. The waiting room of an ND is intended to be a serene place where patients can spend a few minutes in peace and quiet before their consult.

Initial Appointments

An initial appointment with an ND typically lasts about one hour, while follow-up appointments usually last 30 to 60 minutes. During the initial appointment, a detailed medical history is obtained, and a naturopathic assessment is performed. Naturopathic doctors want to have a full understanding of the patient's lifestyle, diet, emotional stressors, current and past symptoms. Their goal is to get a complete picture of how their patient's health issues are related in order to develop the most effective treatment plan for each patient.

Will my naturopathic doctor give me individualized treatment?

As a general rule, naturopathic doctors manage the condition of each one of their patients in a very individualized manner. Even if two patients are diagnosed with the same disorder, they will not necessarily be placed on the same treatment regimen.

The same is true for office visits. The scheduling of follow-up visits varies from one patient to another.

Different patients require different frequencies of follow-up. If a patient feels better after only one or two visits, he may not come back for quite a while. Other patients may require follow-up visits on a weekly basis due to the severity of their illness. Consequently, follow-up visits and treatment plans are tailored to the needs of each patient.

A typical schedule for a new patient might include three appointments within a short period of time to assess his progress as he adopts new protocols for healthy living. During this time, the physician will get to know the patient to determine what he needs to get better, and will help motivate him to consistently implement lifestyle changes. After these initial appointments, the follow-up appointments may then be scheduled on a monthly basis.

How long will it take for me to get results with a naturopathic approach?

The length of time required for patients to experience results after treatment varies due to the nature of their condition, and their ability to comply with their prescribed regimen. Yet patients may start feeling better only a week after their first appointment. However, they should not feel discouraged if positive results take longer to manifest. It may have taken years to develop a given condition, so it is to be expected that it could take several weeks or more to obtain relief.

The nature and speed of the results for each patient partially depends on patients' willingness to make changes in their diet and lifestyle. In some instances, it is necessary for new patients to take very small steps as they find it difficult to give up old habits. On the other hand, there are many patients who are willing to make many changes very quickly. As a general rule, the faster a patient is able to comply with a recommended treatment plan, the more quickly they experience positive results.

Chapter 14

The Best Kept Secret

Patients often ask the question: "If the principles of naturopathic medicine are so obvious (such as reducing stress or having a healthy diet), then why haven't I heard of this before?"

Consider the story of margarine and butter. Many years ago, margarine was advertised as a healthy alternative to butter. People who continued to eat butter were told they were at risk for contracting heart disease. Years later, however, butter was found to have health benefits, while margarine was said to not only be devoid of nutritional value, but also capable of causing detrimental effects on the body.

Now, many years later, despite the numerous studies proving that butter is better than margarine, there are patients coming to naturopathic doctors who eat margarine every day. Clearly, knowledge can become unevenly distributed in our society, perhaps because there are certain organizations that get to choose the kind of information that will be disseminated. For example, the media may focus on merely the latest "health fad" of the times. As a result, important health facts may not reach many patients. Fortunately, naturopathic doctors have a scientific and accurate understanding of health information, which can assure their patients that they are not just jumping on the bandwagon and only following what the media has to offer.

Tips on how to feel and look younger

Many patients discover that they can feel better and younger by simply following some recommendations from their naturopathic doctor. When their pain is reduced, they can acquire a more active lifestyle, lose weight and improve their overall outlook on life.

Sometimes patients ask for natural face creams to make them look younger. Naturopathic doctors may offer very effective facial creams as part of their practice, but to look and feel younger, all that's really necessary is a change in diet. Here are a few key recommendations:

Adopt Healthy Eating Habits

Planning and adopting healthy eating habits is not always easy with the plethora of information sources that vie for our attention. With the right recommendations from an ND, however, many patients develop good eating habits, and as a result, the weight comes off naturally. Weight loss that happens naturally will make patients look and feel younger.

1. Eat Less Sugar

There are studies showing that sugar can cause skin to wrinkle prematurely. Many patients are very surprised to hear this, but many doctors will agree that patients who eat less sugar definitely tend to look younger.

2. Eliminate Dietary Trans-fat

When patients eliminate trans-fat from their diet, and

increase the intake of good oils like olive and coconut oil, they notice that their skin becomes suppler and looks much younger. There is a good reason for this: fats and oils from our diet become part of our cell membranes. To ensure healthy cellular membranes, we need to include a steady stream of "good oils" in our diet.

Trans-fat cannot be considered good oil because it has a very stiff molecular configuration. When it is incorporated into the cell membrane, the membrane becomes less fluid, which affects the appearance of our skin. So, if you want younger-looking skin, eliminate foods containing trans-fats, and take in more coconut and olive oil!

Keep in mind that nutrition and health information is not necessarily common knowledge to everyone, so naturopathic doctors can guide you to make the right decisions. Many NDs will stress the idea that if something is a synthetic substance that was created by man, it may not be the best thing for your body. So, when possible, you want to avoid ingesting such substances.

After implementing recommendations from their naturopathic doctors, patients will often say that they feel many years younger. In addition, if you really want to become healthier, look younger and feel great, the easiest approach may be to do the things that humans have been doing for thousands of years. These include activities like exercising, getting sunlight, drinking water, enjoying life and having fun. All of these things, though seemingly simple, are highly effective in keeping us healthy.

These subtle life changes along with various recommendations from a naturopathic physician, usually transforms patients' lives, causing them to feel so much better overall. It is remarkable how well the body heals when given the right tools.

Chapter 15

There is <u>Always</u> Hope

Is there hope for me?

One of the most wonderful things about naturopathic medicine is that it almost always has a beneficial effect. When a patient applies the principles of natural therapeutics—including regular exercise and a healthy diet replete with nutrients—there is almost always a positive result. There are few cases where naturopathic medicine does not cure the patient. As with traditional medical approaches, there are patients who cannot be completely cured, and patients who are not completely symptom-free, but they can still experience the positive effects of natural medicines without the side effects more common with pharmaceuticals.

There is always hope with naturopathic medicine. No matter what happens to a patient's health, there is always some form of naturopathic treatment that can help.

There are countless natural ways to heal the body. If a patient has the motivation to make the necessary changes and the commitment to persist in implementing those changes, the results can be nothing short of amazing.

Naturopathic medicine has helped desperate patients who strongly believed that their illness was life-threatening or incurable because they were told by main stream medicine that nothing could be done to help them. For example, even patients who were told they could never conceive may now be able to have children despite experiencing many different surgeries and severe endometriosis in the past.

Naturopathic medicine is an amazing system of healing that *works*. It enables people to make major changes and transform their lives. All they need is hope and a willingness to try.

Embrace the possibilities that are available to you each and every day to make healthy, natural choices. The healing will manifest; with the right guidance it can happen!

Articles by Dr. Finker

Cancer Fighting Foods

Dietary intake provides a foundation for the human body to be healthy. Foods can either support and nourish the body or potentially cause harm. The incidence of developing cancer is extremely high; one person out of three will have some form of cancer in their lifetime.

Fortunately, there are many things that can be done to help prevent cancer. Eating foods that have been proven to have cancer fighting benefits can potentially save lives. These foods will have even more potent anti-cancer agents if you make sure that they are organic.

Organic foods are higher in vitamins and minerals, which help to decrease the risk of cancer. Also, diets that include large amounts of vegetables have been shown to fight off cancer. Thus, it is important that the following specific foods along with many vegetables are included in our daily diets.

Drink Organic Green Tea

One of the most well studied foods is actually a drink that decreases cancer risk: green tea. Green tea has been used for thousands of years and has many cancer fighting properties. It contains antioxidants, which help to prevent damage to cells, so it is protective against cancer. Bladder cancer, breast cancer, and even skin cancer have been shown to be helped by green tea.

Some studies show that just three cups of tea a day can reduce the risk of breast cancer in young women.

Research shows that the chances of developing a breast cancer tumor drop by around 37 percent in women under 50 who drank tea at least three times daily. Other studies have shown that women of all ages would benefit from drinking eight cups of green tea daily to prevent breast cancer. Green tea also modulates blood sugar levels. High blood sugar levels have been linked with increased cancer risk. Green tea is one of the best super-foods to ward off cancer as long as it's fluoride free.

Eat Organic Blueberries

Blueberries are a very tasty way to help ward off cancer. The antioxidants in blueberries called anthocyanins have been shown to prevent cancer and specifically to reduce colon cancer risk. Several studies have demonstrated that blueberries decrease the risk of metastases, which is a cancer spreading from its original site. Blueberries are low on the glycemic index so they usually do not affect sugar levels like other fruits can. Eating a cup of wild blueberries a day can help to prevent cancer.

Mushrooms for Immunity

Many mushrooms contain compounds that can help the body fight cancer. Shitake, maitake, reishi, and even the inexpensive button mushrooms all have immune boosting properties, which help prevent cancer. Reishi mushrooms have been shown to inhibit the growth of malignant tumors. Maitake mushrooms may help reduce blood sugar levels, which will reduce cancer risk. Mushrooms can be high in pesticides and thus it is best to eat organic mushrooms.

Eat Your Vegetables

Cruciferous vegetables such as broccoli, cauliflower, cabbage, brussel sprouts, bok choy, kale, etc. have been shown to help decrease the risk of cancer, especially breast cancer. Cruciferous vegetables have been shown to contain DIM (diindolylmethane) and I3C (Indole-3-Carbinol). Indole-3-carbinol is a phytonutrient which is an organic plant part specifically found in cruciferous vegetables. Other phytonutrients that we may be more familiar with include carotenoids, which are the red, yellow and orange pigments in vegetables. DIM is also a phytonutrient that is a break down product of Indole-3-Carbinol. These two phytonutrients help to convert bad estrogen over to good estrogen. I3C has been shown to be very effective in fighting breast cancer cells by blocking tumor growth. Research has shown that both I3C and DIM may potentially even help cure cancer.

Eat Garlic

Garlic is an important food that helps to fight cancer. Garlic contains a powerful plant phytonutrient called allicin that has been shown to protect the body against cancer. Allicin has even been shown to kill tumor cells in certain studies. Garlic can have a powerful antioxidant effect in the body, which means it helps to protect against damaging free radicals, which can cause cancer. Studies have found that high consumption of raw or cooked garlic decreases the risk of colon cancer and stomach cancer by up to 50%.

Green tea, blueberries, mushrooms, cruciferous vegetables, and garlic are very potent anti-cancer foods and everyone would benefit from adding these foods to their diet. There are many other foods that are not listed here that would help as well. In general, ingesting the super foods listed above along with a lot of organic vegetables will help to minimize your risk of developing cancer.

Infertility and Getting Pregnant Naturally

It is difficult to determine a woman's ability to become pregnant and sometimes it doesn't follow along the doctor's prognosis. Patients who are diagnosed as infertile for long periods of time with no underlying known cause may only have a simple nutritional deficiency. For example, these patients may have been deficient in zinc and when zinc was administered, they were able to conceive.

Some of the most common reasons why women experience infertility are stress, hormone imbalances and nutritional deficiencies. It's commonplace for women to have difficulty conceiving for years but then easily become pregnant after they adopt a child. This happens because once the pressure to have children is removed, couples can relax and are able to have children naturally. Normalizing patients' adrenal glands, balancing their hormones and healing their nutritional deficiencies often facilitates pregnancy.

However, there are also patients who have complicated cases. They could have endometriosis, ovarian cysts or other medical conditions. Some of these women are told they are never going to be able to conceive. Sometimes these patients can work really hard changing their diet and taking supplements and then despite the dismal prognosis, become pregnant.

Stress and Infertility

Relaxation is a very important step that can help women become pregnant. Often women are stressed out because they are not getting pregnant. Stress automatically increases their cortisol levels and decreases the pregnancy hormone progesterone. This was important in ancient times when people had to deal with conditions of famine.

It was important to disrupt the pregnancy process under times of stress so that mother and baby would not starve to death. However, in modern times, stressors such as traffic and busy work schedules can cause unnecessary problems with infertility. These women could benefit from practicing daily relaxation techniques from tai chi to yoga.

Diet, Hormones and Fertility

Diet either helps or hinders fertility. Diets lacking in nutrients can alter fertility. Patients on a processed food diet can switch over to whole foods, and then have an easier time conceiving. Also, taking various supplements to help support the body under the guidance of a doctor can help women become pregnant.

A common dietary ingredient that has been scientifically shown to decrease fertility is processed soy. Soy decreases sperm count as well as hinders women's ability to get pregnant by disrupting their hormone balance. Dairy and beef products that have growth hormones can also cause imbalances with female hormones.

IVF and Other Fertility Drugs

In certain circumstances, patients can become very sick from IVF and other fertility drugs. In some cases this can even cause hospitalization. However, these same patients can undergo IVF treatment in adjunct with natural medicine and have favorable outcomes. IVF treatments should only be used as a last resort and always should be combined with supportive natural medicine. Fortunately, there are many vitamins, botanicals and lifestyle changes that can help patients become pregnant naturally without the use of IVF and other fertility drugs.

Canola Oil is Not a Health Food

Despite popular belief, canola oil is not good for us. It is hard to understand this because in most health food stores canola oil is a staple ingredient. Today, almost all types of canola oil (rapeseed oil) are considered a genetically modified organism or GMO.

This type of food alteration is alarming and should be avoided at all costs. GMO's are created by transferring the gene from one species such as viruses, bacteria, or animals into the DNA of another species such as the canola seed. This sounds like science fiction, but GMO's are in many of the foods that we consume. Most consumers (75%) are completely unaware of this due to the absence of labeling.

The malevolent health effects from GMO foods shown in animal testing include: allergic reactions, gastrointestinal problems, and even death. It has even been shown that animals will avoid GMO foods when given an alternative. There are no human studies, but workers on GMO farms suffer from severe allergies. Also, I have observed in my practice that patients with severe gastrointestinal discomfort heal solely from avoiding these foods.

The literature is mixed on the health virtues of the non-GMO organic canola oil including both positive and some scary health information. However, it is difficult to distinguish between the organic canola oil and the GMO version. Thus, it is in our best interest to avoid canola oil and other GMO foods.

There are so many oils that are good for us, that have been used for centuries, so avoid canola oil and escape potential health problems.

Health Benefits of Raw Honey

One of the oldest sweeteners known to man is raw organic honey.

Raw honey eaten in small doses can be quite beneficial for the body. This differs from the processed honey that we are used to consuming which is similar to regular sugar and should be avoided.

Also, only consume organic raw honey ensuring that the bees have not been fed high fructose corn syrup and that no pesticides were used in the process. This affects the quality of the honey and there has been a correlation between pesticides and high fructose corn syrup administration in threatening the very existence of the honey bee.

Raw honey is great for the body because it contains enzymes, antioxidants, vitamins, and minerals that are not found in processed honey. It helps to balance good gastrointestinal bacteria and can even lower homocysteine levels decreasing heart disease risk. Also there has been some clinical evidence showing that eating local raw honey can help with allergies.

Believe it or not, raw honey can even be used topically to help to heal wounds! So much so that honey has even been used for wound healing in the hospital setting due to its antimicrobial properties. It also works great as a natural face mask to help decrease inflammation associated with dry skin and acne.

Where to find this amazing natural cure-all? Locally cultivated raw organic honey can be found at your local health-food store.

5 Easy Steps to Reduce Anxiety

Anxiety has become a very common health problem that is often treated with various medications. Although pharmaceuticals can be effective, they are not treating the underlying cause of the problem which can be as simple as sleep deprivation.

Here are 5 simple steps that you can take to help decrease anxiety:

1. First, sleep between eight and nine hours in order to help balance your stress hormones.

2. Keep the bedroom completely dark to ensure a good night sleep which elevates feel good hormones like melatonin.

3. Eat a snack or meal during the day every three to four hours that contains protein. This will help to maintain optimum blood sugar levels which will help to balance stress hormones.

4. It is important to avoid stimulants such as chocolate and coffee especially after 3:00 p.m. because it will increase stress hormones and disrupt the circadian rhythm.

5. Most importantly, incorporate some kind of exercise into your daily routine. Exercise helps to normalize the stress response and can be very effective in treating anxiety. Employing some kind of daily moving relaxation techniques such as yoga or tai chi also helps to decrease anxiety levels.

In addition to the above techniques, the underlying causes of anxiety can be helped with nutrition, herbs, vitamins, and so on to bring the body back into balance allowing us to relax and once again have a sense of well-being. There are various blood tests and other means of testing that can determine what deficiencies your body has. Your doctor can then prescribe supplements to help heal the underlying causes of your anxiety.

Note: *Please seek the guidance from your doctor to determine which supplements would be appropriate for you.*

The Risk of Mold Exposure

Indoor mold is a health hazard that is relatively commonplace in many homes and buildings. According to the CDC mold can grow on anything as long as there is moisture in the air.

Mold has been known to cause health problems since ancient man. In fact, in biblical times if a dwelling was continuously moldy it was condemned and torn down. Molds give off a poisonous substance called mycotoxins which can cause a variety of health problems ranging from an allergic response to neurological problems.

Symptoms of mold exposure include but are not limited to: asthma, sinus infections, tremors, memory loss, numbness and tingling, and muscle weakness. Also, mold exposure as an infant has been linked to multiple allergy risk later on in life.

Unfortunately, mold contamination is so prevalent that mold exposure in the home is estimated to be the cause of 4.6 million cases of asthma per year in the USA. If mold is a problem in the home it is very important to remove it as soon as possible and then prevent it from re-growing.

In order to prevent health problems and a costly clean up, it is always best to prevent mold from growing by being proactive and to install an air monitoring system to have timely information on air quality.

All of the health problems associated with mold are treatable. Asthma, sinus infections, etc. are all helped through dietary changes, supplementation, and avoidance of further mycotoxin exposure.

Secrets to Avoiding the Flu... Naturally

The flu virus has gotten a lot of attention over the years from the media. Many people are extremely anxious about catching the flu. Fortunately there are several ways to prevent the flu by maintaining a strong immune system and by practicing good hygiene.

One simple way to prevent infection is by washing your hands with regular soap before touching your eyes or eating food. The main way disease spreads is through our mucous membranes. The best way to prevent pathogens from getting into the body is by washing your hands thoroughly with regular soap.

Antibacterial soap and hand sanitizers have been shown to create superbugs and pathogens that our bodies are not familiar with; even the CDC feels that using these products are "cause for concern." Regular soap kills germs effectively and does not create superbugs.

Vitamin D has been proven to prevent the onset of the flu virus. Thus, it is very important to make sure that your vitamin D levels are within normal range. Make sure that your doctor is testing your vitamin D levels with the 25-Hydroxy-Vitamin-D test and then prescribes the required dose of vitamin D to prevent infection.

Adequate sleep, a healthy diet, and keeping stress levels low have been shown to boost the immune system and will help ward off the flu. In addition to Vitamin D there are other supplements that prevent flu onset such as: vitamin C, echinacea, elderberry, etc. Please seek the guidance from your doctor to determine which supplements would be appropriate for you.

The Truth about Vitamin D Deficiency

Because most of us live in cold climates that cause us to stay indoors most of the day, many people are deficient in Vitamin D especially during the winter months.

Vitamin D deficiency can cause problems such as fractures, osteoporosis, and psoriasis. Also fibromyalgia-like symptoms: muscle pain, muscle weakness and bone pain may be caused by vitamin D deficiency. It can also cause more serious health problems such as increased risk for cancer; such as breast and colon cancer.

Some of us even avoid the sun during the summer months, which may help to prevent the least invasive form of skin cancer, basal cell carcinoma; however, it causes us to be vulnerable to many other problems. In fact studies show that patients who develop basal cell carcinoma are at a decreased risk for developing colon cancer.

The best way to increase the body's levels of Vitamin D is through sun exposure, at least 30% of a person's skin surface for 30 minutes at moderate latitudes. It is important not to burn and to consult your doctor before exposing yourself to the sun if you are on any medications that may increase the risk of sunburn. Cod liver oil, sardines, egg yolks and mushrooms are good food sources of Vitamin D.

Of course, always make sure to consult your doctor before taking any kind of cod liver oil or synthetic Vitamin D. Your doctor can monitor your blood levels of Vitamin D (25-OH Vitamin D) and then supplement with food, sun exposure and Vitamin D3 (cholecalciferol) if applicable.

Article about Dr. Finker

How to Make Buying Organic Affordable

Source: *OrganicAuthority.com*

Dr. Jillian Finker is definitely biased when it comes to eating organic foods.

"I have always been an advocate for organic foods, including baby foods," the naturopathic doctor from Bellmore New York, tells OrganicAuthority.com. "I was brought up on organic baby food, I always purchase organic products, and I recommend that my patients eat organic food whenever possible."

Dr. Finker's professional experience has reaffirmed her commitment to the organic lifestyle.

"I have personally seen patients whose lives have been ruined by their exposure to pesticides," she says. "Their bodies were loaded with pesticides from either spray exposure or from ingesting heavily sprayed fruits and vegetables. These patients have a variety of symptoms, ranging from paresthesia (a sensation of burning, prickling, itching, or tingling, with no apparent physical cause) to skin rashes. It saddens me that we still use pesticides on our foods, even though there are organic farming options available to us."

It's hard to argue with Dr. Finker's logic, unless you work for a nonorganic food manufacturer whose products are laced with pesticides. But ask average consumers about eating organically, and one issue seems to emerge universally: "It's too expensive."

Wrong.

Eating organically needn't be a wallet buster, says Debra Stark, owner of Debra's Natural Gourmet, a retail store in Concord, Massachusetts. Buying organic beans, grains, pasta, herbs, spices, leafy greens and other produce is not only economical, but far healthier than plunking down a few bucks for a prepackaged meal that contains only one nutritionally questionable serving.

"There are times when our organic fruits and veggies cost less than commercially grown ones in the supermarket," Stark tells OrganicAuthority.com. "But even when they don't, there are always items that are affordable. Besides, look at the bottom line: A commercially grown head of romaine, for instance, is subsidized by the government. By the time we all pay for the damage to the environment that the chemical fertilizers, herbicides and pesticides wreak-the extra health-care costs incurred by farm workers because of their exposure to the toxic-stuff a regular head of romaine costs each of us over $3.50. I saw these figures some years ago from the U.S. Department of Agriculture. Organic farmers receive no subsidies, and last week our organic romaine was $1.49 per head."

And the price gap between nonorganic and organic foods continues to narrow.

"Whenever economies of scale come into play, prices go down," Stark says. "With big players entering the natural products industry, many products like cold cereals, for instance, are being produced on a larger scale."

Another source for economical organic foods is farmers' markets.

"They're great fun," Stark says. "They allow us to meet the people who work hard growing our food. Even if that head of lettuce costs more than the tired head sitting in the supermarket, the value is greater. Just think how many more vitamins and minerals there are in a fresh, just-picked-that-morning head of lettuce than in the one that had to travel across country. There's better all-over nutrient value-and it's also better value from the standpoint of the community. Local farmers pay local taxes and make contributions to local schools. It all depends, you see, on how we define value."

"Consumers find reasonably priced organic products the same way they find reasonably priced anything: They do their homework and read," adds herbalist Melinda Olson, owner of Tualatin, Oregon-based Earth Mama Angel Baby, a producer of natural and organic products for pregnancy, labor, postpartum recovery, breastfeeding and baby care. "More and more, organic products are finding their way into mainstream retail stores alongside conventional products," she tells *OrganicAuthority.com*, "and new grocery chains are 'sneaking' organics in, under the guise of being trendy."

Read labels to get more organic "bang for your buck," she advises. "The biggest question to examine is: What makes a product 'reasonably-priced'? In my opinion, paying a little bit more, in order to avoid ingesting or applying herbicides, pesticides, chemical fertilizers, hormones and antibiotics, makes the purchase more than 'reasonable.' I'd say that makes it a very valuable and cost-effective purchase indeed."

"Price is not an issue because I decided it would not be," says holistic health counselor Cynthia Stadd of New York City.

"I am aware that I spend more on food bills than I used to, but I see it as prevention from spending tons more on doctors' bills and medications," she tells OrganicAuthority. com. "I see organic food as one tool to sustaining vibrant health, without the need for doctors."

What Dr. Finker's Patients are Saying…

I first went to see Dr. Finker two years ago when I was diagnosed with Hypothyroidism, a condition stemming from Hashimoto's disease. I made a decision that I did not want to be on Synthroid the rest of my life so I went to Dr. Finker.

She corrected my thyroid in eight weeks!

Granted, I was and still am on a strict diet and supplements, but my thyroid is now functioning as it should and I feel fantastic.

Since then, I have seen Dr. Finker for ongoing health wellness and most recently brought my daughter in due to fluid in her ears. She had fluid in her ears for two months and the ENT wanted to put tubes in, of course. I took her to Dr. Finker and in three weeks her ears are now clear of fluid. No surgery needed. I am a happy mom with an even happier daughter!

But my praises are not only because she helped both my daughter and I. Most of my praises are for Dr. Finker's uniqueness.

She is extremely knowledgeable and takes a holistic approach to healing. She wants to make sure your whole body is in balance, not just quickly fix the one thing of concern at that moment. She is also patient and really takes the time to listen to all your concerns and questions and will never make you feel like you are wasting her time. I also love that she always takes the most conservative approach to healing first. She makes every effort to get your body back on track through diet changes or homeopathic remedies. She does not push supplements on you, unless really necessary.

Above all, she is the most compassionate doctor I have met. Her desire to heal her patients is her passion and it is obvious by her demeanor, concern and empathy.

I am eternally grateful for all she has done for our family thus far and she will always be the first one I call with any major health issues.

With great appreciation,

—*Francine S., North Carolina*

I started seeing Dr. Finker after having four months of symptoms like anxiety, depression, blurred vision, nervousness, jittery feelings, phobias and fears.

Every doctor I went to over that time diagnosed me with anxiety and recommended that I try antidepressants or Benzo's. I did not feel this was the way I wanted to go and more importantly I felt there was more to it than that. My family also felt this way because both of my parents had actually dealt with low blood sugar when they were younger and had many of the same symptoms so I was pretty sure I needed to see a doctor that knew how to treat it and there aren't many around.

I found her name reading an article out of *Woman's World* about hypoglycemia and how to treat it. I never had any issues with anything like this in the past. As soon as I saw Dr. Finker, she said we would get to the bottom of this so I could start feeling better. After doing some tests and hearing my symptoms we found out my cortisol was very high as well as my hormones and I had low blood sugar.

Dr. Finker put me on a very specific diet regimen as well as exercise and supplements to take with every meal.

After a few months I started to feel much better and now it is 10 months later and I'm almost back to myself. I am so happy that I found Dr. Finker because I wanted to get to the root of the problem and solve it the natural way rather than being drugged up on med's for the rest of my life. Not only do I feel better now but I also lost about 40 lbs. and I just feel that I am so much healthier in general. For me, Dr. Finker really helped me get my life back on track from a very tough time and I think she is wonderful!

—*Jen S., Long Island*

Dr. Finker has the unique ability, unlike many traditional doctors these days, to take the time to get to know her patients' lifestyles, habits, likes and dislikes. This interest translates into a genuine concern for their well being, and the ability to recommend changes, prescribe vitamins and supplements, advise on healthy eating habits and inspire them to make positive "whole life" adjustments.

I sought Dr. Finker's advice after numerous doctors and traditional medical tests could not locate the reason behind the abdominal pain which I was experiencing for months, in addition to feeling run-down and lethargic. After following her advice for one week, I discovered that I had an intolerance for certain foods (soy) that was literally making me sick and bloated.

Now after almost one year of following the guidelines that she suggested, I am pain-free, have tripled my energy level, have lost weight and feel terrific... and unlike many women my age (56), I am not on any type of medication for any physical issues!! I will continue to consult with Dr. Finker in the future because she is a wealth of information and I personally feel I can ask her advice on any topic.

—*Jan Y., Florida*

I have been treated by Dr. Finker for about a year. Dr. Finker was able to diagnose and treat my body using changes in my lifestyle along with natural minerals, glandulars, and vitamins. It has worked out wonderfully and those changes have balanced me out which no else was able to do.

Dr. Finker is a non-judgmental, caring individual and anyone can work with her and get good results. She has treated a lot of different issues and will do her research to find out what will help you.

Yes… I would recommend everyone to work with Dr. Finker… she is the best.

—*Sharon W., Long Island*

Dear Dr. Finker,

I started with you approximately two years ago and I just wanted to thank you for all of your help. I had gone to my regular M.D.'S and was advised because I am diabetic for over 20 years, I was starting to develop kidney failure and there was nothing I could do about it. My back was always hurting me and I worried about my kidney becoming diseased. The kidney failure was beginning to show in my urine. I had also gone to my endocrinologist, very upset that there were no vitamins or supplements to stop this from happening. I did not want to go on dialysis.

After coming to your office, you told me that you could help. I started taking Renal plus, and coenzyme kd. I removed all beef from my diet as well as all white products. After taking the products and diet recommendations, I took another urine test six months later and my problem had gone away.

I am very grateful that I will not have to go on kidney dialysis since the kidney problem I had did not progress to a point where it went into my blood or needed further drastic conventional treatment.

For the above reason, I recommend you to everyone I speak with. I appreciate your time, knowledge and professionalism. My regular M.D.'s don't understand how I reversed my lab numbers.

Sincerely,

—Debbie T., Long Island

Dr. Finker was one of the best gifts I gave to myself. My first consultation with her happened to be on my 50th birthday. From our first meeting I remember sharing a perceptive chuckle! She is understanding and intuitive. I know the "stars" brought us together. I'm a native New Yorker living in Bermuda for almost 15 years. I was researching for a naturopathic doctor on Long Island.

I felt a tug toward Dr. Finker but I must confess she was not the first N.D. I pursued online. Gratefully, I was quickly deterred from my initial choice and went with my gut feeling (as we should always do) and contacted Dr. Finker. My concern at the time was menopause and the unwelcoming symptoms, besides wanting to live naturally and make alternative medical choices. At the initial consultation, Dr. Finker recommended supplements and needless to say she was right on target. The results of my blood work and hormone panel, once received, proved Dr. Finker's recommendations true to the tee!

That was over seven years ago and all I can say is that every consultation is a testimonial. For each ailment or complaint, Dr. Finker's expert health care provided improvement and healing. Dr. Finker provides so much support in so many ways. Not just physical, but emotional and spiritual. She always seems to know just what to say and in the fewest words you know she reads your email, understands it, and encourages you. Dr. Finker is caring, inspiring and generous. She always makes me feel better. So much so that I have booked consultations at times because I was feeling down, lethargic, emotionally drained and facing personal problems at their climax. The minute we consulted, her energy just seemed to melt away my issues so that I had to stop and think 'what is bothering me'?!!

Over the years, my experience is that Dr. Finker's health care is very personalized and she has helped me, through supplements, therapy and kindness, overcome menopausal symptoms, abnormal tiredness, weight gain and emotional traumas, to achieve my personal best. The précis of my testimony is that Dr. Finker makes me believe I can achieve my youthful physique, stamina and physical, emotional and spiritual best. 'I don't know what I would do without Dr. Finker'! She is a true BLESSING.

—Adrienne G., Bermuda

I first met Dr. Finker when I took my teenage daughter to her for general anxiety disorder. Dr. Finker was very understanding and helpful. She put my daughter and I at ease with her gentle manner. She put her on a program that was easy enough to follow, and it worked wonders. I am happy to say her anxiety is behind her! We credit Dr. Finker's knowledge and kindness.

—Leanora K., Long Island

Dr. Finker is the consummate professional... a compassionate, knowledgeable practitioner who provides her wise guidance and uncommonly good sense to support my intuitive approach to self care. When I first sought

Dr. Finker's expertise, I needed relief from overwhelming adrenal and thyroid symptoms which depleted my energy, focus and ability to function. The personalized, comprehensive plan of care she recommended incorporated diet, exercise, lifestyle modifications and natural therapies to restore my health and wellbeing.

As a nurse educator for nearly 30 years, I truly value Dr. Finker's balanced approach and keen insight as she combines art and science to empower and partner with her patients, gently guiding them toward overall wellness.

—Mona G., RN,FNP, Long Island

Dr. Finker was the first naturopathic doctor I had to see. She listened carefully to my health challenge and guided me back to health with helpful advice and quality nutritional supplements. I would highly recommend her to family and friends with their health challenges.

—Anthony T., Long Island

Prior to seeing Dr. Finker, my periods had always been irregular. I spent three miserable years on Yasmin, tolerating the insufferable mood swings and debilitating physical side effects—all because I blindly trusted my gynecologist and his endorsement of what he seemed to claim was some sort of miracle tablet.

Ultimately, I realized that no one had ever identified the CAUSE of my menstrual irregularities. According to every doctor I'd ever seen, my blood-work indicated that my hormone levels were "normal." Frustrated and concerned, I considered consulting a naturopathic physician. I got Dr. Finker's name and contact information from a friend whom she has also helped tremendously.

Unlike practitioners of standard, Western medicine, Dr. Finker is a holistic health practitioner, recognizing that no part of the body is isolated in a vacuum—everything is connected to everything else! Likewise, Dr. Finker recognizes that each patient's body is different; therefore, she custom-designs a schedule/list of suggestions for each individual patient.

Dr. Finker identified the underlying causes of my menstrual irregularities and helped me to get my body back on track through diet, vitamin supplements, and bio-identical (as opposed to synthetic) hormones. She is a knowledgeable, compassionate, and reassuring physician; I am infinitely thankful to have found her!

—Anonymous, New York

About Dr. Finker

Dr. Finker, Naturopathic Doctor, is a primary care doctor who is an expert in alternative medicine. She combines the latest scientific information along with natural therapeutics that have been used effectively for centuries, in order to provide individualized treatments for all of her patients. Dr. Finker compassionately guides all of her patients back onto their path of well-being. "There is always hope," she says. "There are many places to seek help; the possibilities are endless."

Dr. Finker specializes in women's health, helping females with various hormonal problems ranging from PMS to infertility. Dr. Finker is an expert when it comes to helping patients with thyroid issues, gastrointestinal problems and anxiety. She utilizes nutrition, supplements, homeopathy and various other healing techniques to help heal her patients' health problems.

Dr. Finker has a medical clinic in Connecticut, along with her private practice in Bellmore, New York. She specializes in women's health and is an expert in natural medicine. Dr. Finker was selected as the "Best Alternative Doctor on Long Island" for 2011, 2012 and 2013. She has appeared on various television programs and acts as a consultant for several international companies. Her work has been featured in various books and major magazines nationwide. Visit her website at: *www.drfinker.com*

Notes

Notes

Notes